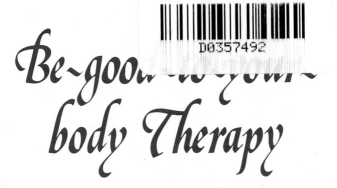

Be-good-to-your body Therapy

Be-good-to-your-body Therapy

written by
Steve Ilg

illustrated by
R.W. Alley

ONE
CARING
PLACE

Abbey Press

Text © 1992 Steve Ilg
Illustrations © 1992 St. Meinrad Archabbey
Published by One Caring Place
Abbey Press
St. Meinrad, Indiana 47577

Library of Congress Catalog Number
92-73686

ISBN 0-87029-255-2

Printed in the United States of America

Foreword

As we travel paths of personal growth and transformation, we often overlook a vital component that comes along on the journey—our bodies!

Yet the way we physically experience life cannot be separated from our spiritual and psychological reality. How we feel in our bodies has an impact on our entire being. And, conversely, what the heart and the soul know of bliss and pain reverberates through each cell.

Be-good-to-your-body Therapy demonstrates that a fitness program involves more than jumping in an exercise class or lifting weights at the gym. Its holistic approach incorporates strength training, kinesthetic movement, cardiovascular activity, nutrition, and meditation. Grounded in accepting, loving, and respecting the body, it points the way to developing inner power and a more intense appreciation for living.

With the guidelines in *Be-good-to-your-body Therapy*, you can experience your workout sessions as moments when you touch the incredible God-given magnificence that flows and radiates within you. And the physical fitness you attain will truly be a natural expression of your inner joy.

1.

Your body is a masterpiece, intricate in function, unique in its mix of attributes and abilities. Give praise—you are wonderfully, singularly made!

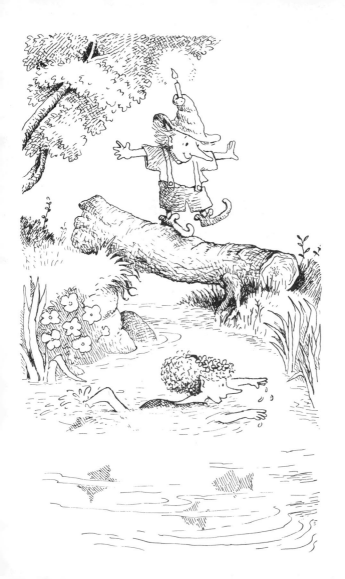

2.

The cells of your body are composed of matter recycled since the beginning of the universe. You are stardust— let your light shine!

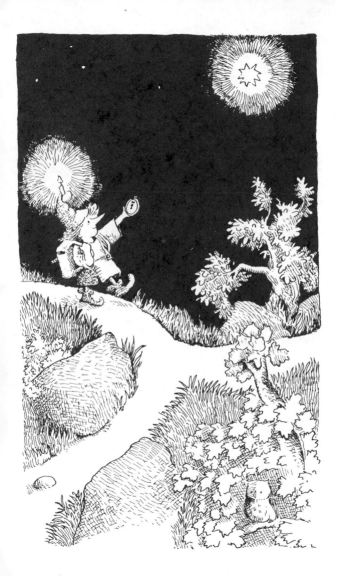

3.

Your body is beautiful just as it is. It need not measure up to imposed standards of beauty. What's important is how your body looks and feels and works according to you.

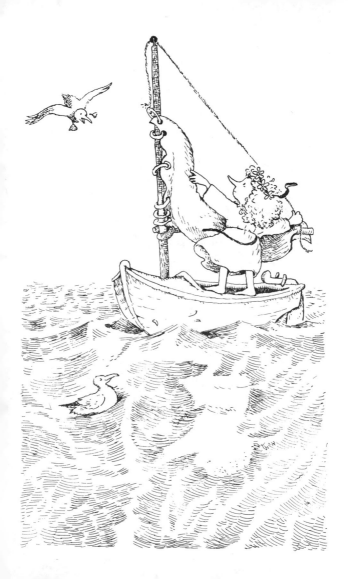

4.

If you're unhappy with some part of your physical self, dialogue with it. Listen to the wisdom of your body.

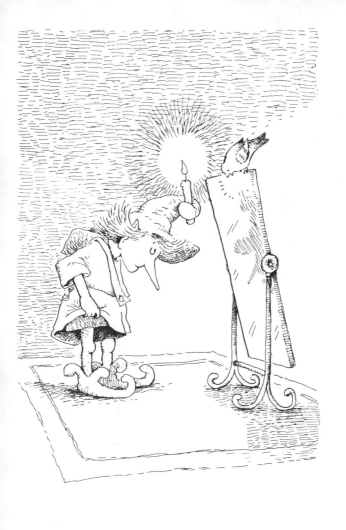

5.

To exist within a body is a magnificent gift from God. Keeping fit honors the sacredness of that gift.

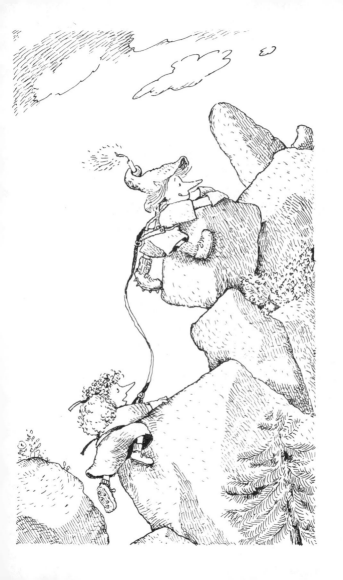

6.

A fitness program is not punishment for an imperfect body, but a sign of care. Love your body as it is. Then act to keep it well-suited to the life tasks to which you are called.

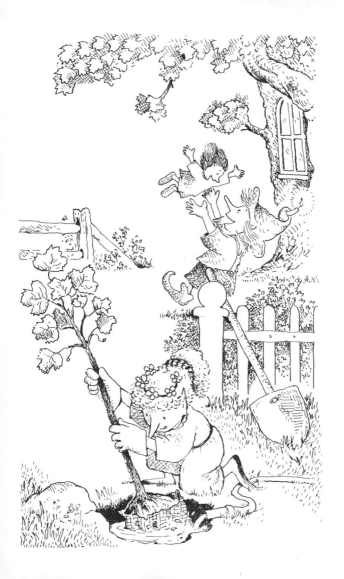

7.

Take from fitness guides what your heart is attracted to, and let the rest go. Picture how you want your body to look; imagine how you wish to feel. Your mind will steer your body toward your goal; your heart will provide the fuel.

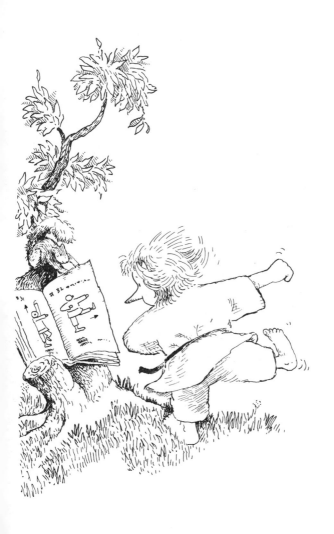

8.

Fitness training is a journey; establish your own unique route. With overtraining, or "too much too soon," you can lose interest. Begin slowly, and progress at your own pace.

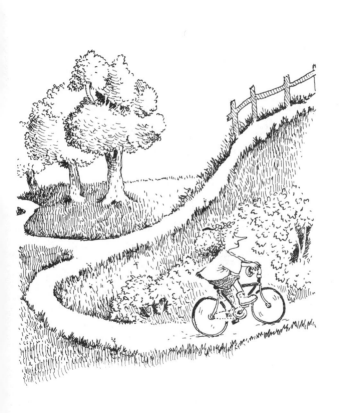

9.

Take a cleansing breath, notice how the world breathes with you, and relax. Relaxing lets you perform more smoothly, efficiently, beautifully.

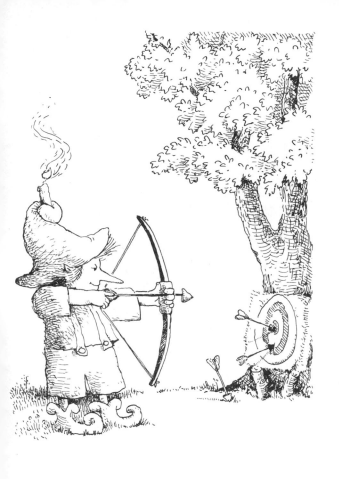

10.

Present a graceful posture to
the world; awaken your spine.
Pretend your head is suspended
from above. An awakened spine
sends joy and energy throughout
your body.

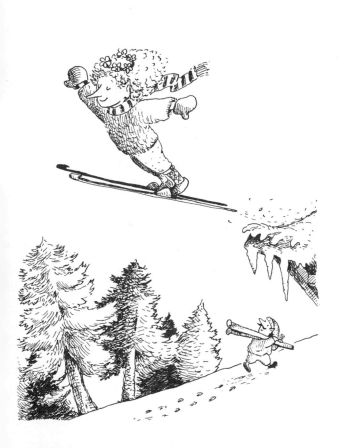

11.

Include strength training in your fitness plan. This keeps your joints strong and develops inner power. You achieve unity of breath, posture, and mental focus.

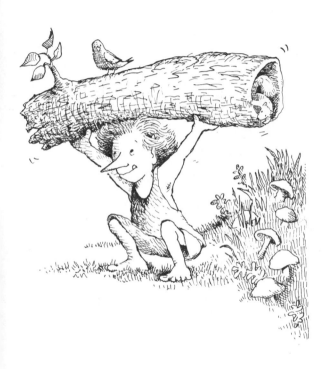

12.

Do kinesthetic activity—like stretching, dance, gymnastics. This teaches you how to be supple and move gracefully. You breathe more softly; you walk more intuitively with the earth.

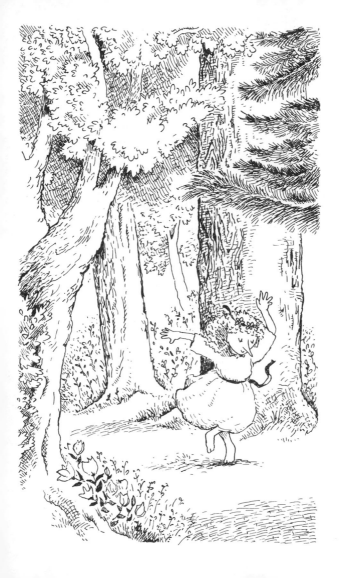

13.

Use cardiovascular activity to empower your heart and lungs and maintain an efficient body weight appropriate for you. This teaches you patience, rhythm, and perseverance.

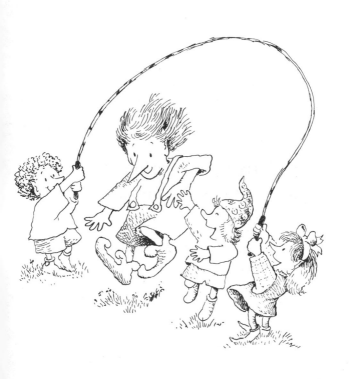

14.

Be attentive to nutrition. Your body is fashioned from earth, and from the earth's harvest it draws well-being. Listen to your body; it will tell you what it needs.

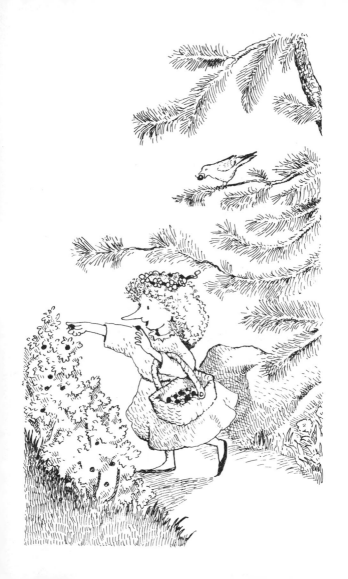

15.

Have quiet times in your fitness program. Meditation fuses your inner and outer selves, making you one with your body. It allows you to receive and experience the Divine Presence.

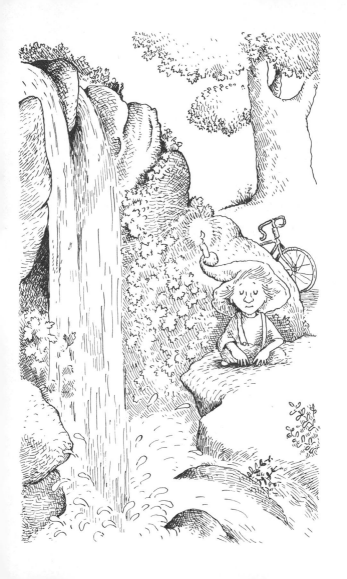

16.

When you're feeling overwhelmed, do strength training. You'll feel more centered; your spirit will become more radiant.

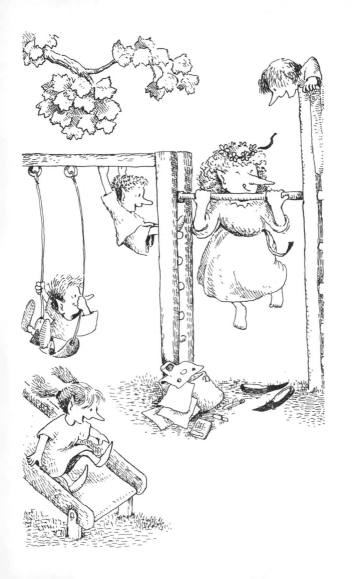

17.

When you feel tight, constricted, or ungraceful, do stretching, dancing, or some other kinesthetic activity. Soon you will regain your breath, your posture, and your natural elegance.

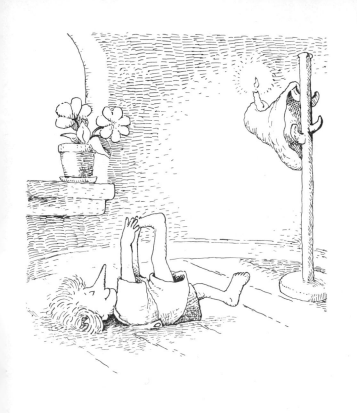

18.

When you're angry or restless, go for a run, a bike ride, or a walk. Feel the tempo of your breathing within the rhythm of nature.

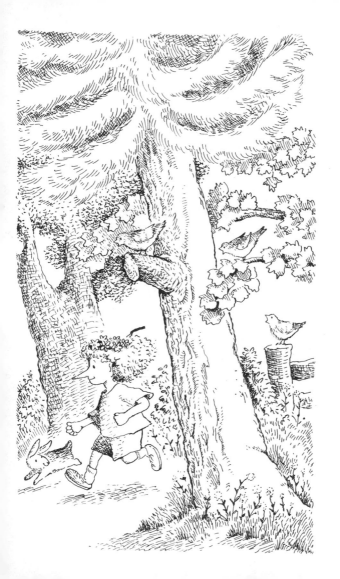

19.

When you feel irritable or tired, consider your nutrition. What you eat directly affects how you feel and perform. Eat gently when you feel anxious; eat strongly when you feel weak.

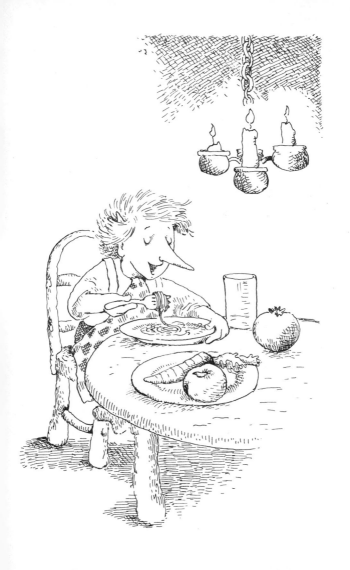

20.

When worries seem to be crushing you, take some meditative moments to appreciate the wonder of your own life experience. Know that you are exactly where you need to be.

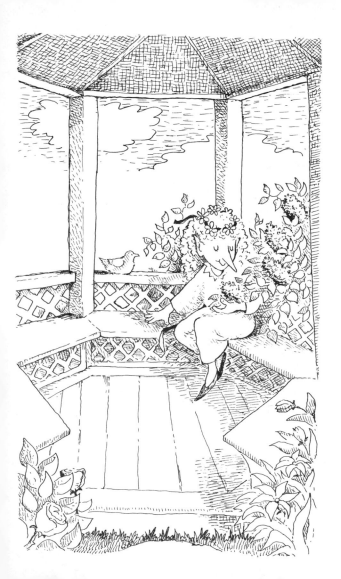

21.

Self-congratulation is a necessary form of communication with your body. Reward yourself for your fitness efforts. Positive transformations need encouragement.

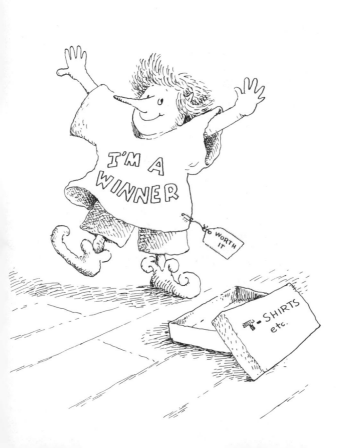

22.

Nothing has power over your fitness training unless you give it power. Approach difficulties with a light spirit. Renew your intentions when you feel dejected. Look excuses in the eye, and gently toss them from your path. This is known as will power.

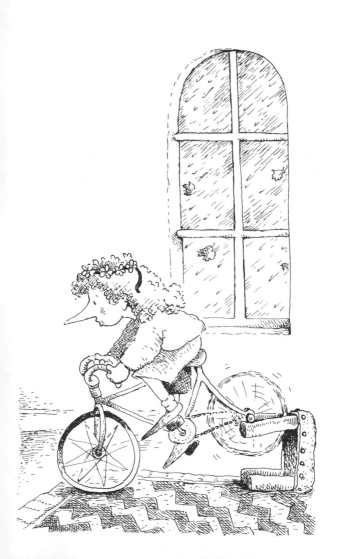

23.

Don't fear changes in your body or in your attitude; change is essential. Seek small changes, not big end points.

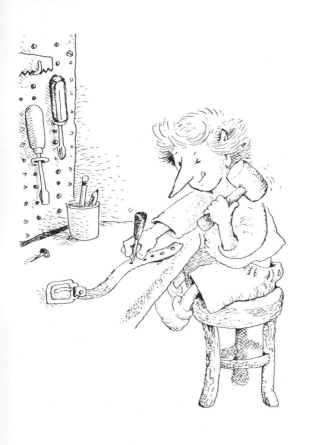

24.

Welcome family and friends to share your workouts. They help unfold your enjoyment and progress.

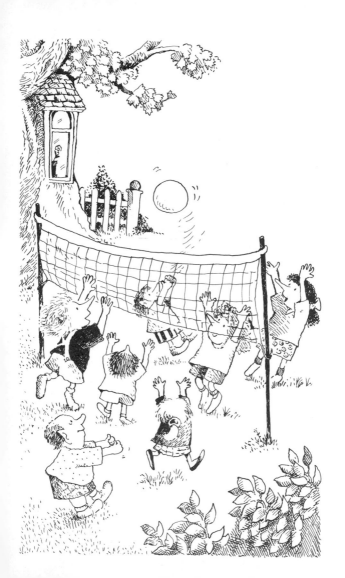

25.

Work out with animals, especially pets. Study how they move. They are true fitness masters and love to teach.

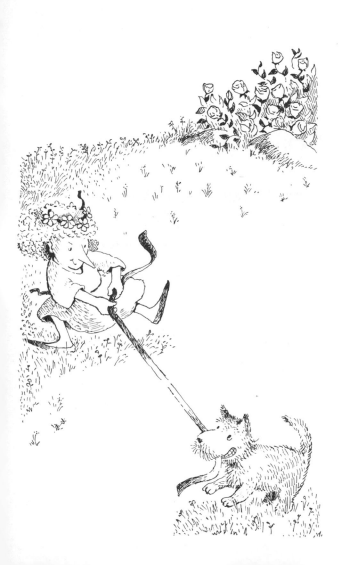

26.

Have a friend photograph you doing something physical that you enjoy. Notice how energetic and free-flowing you look.

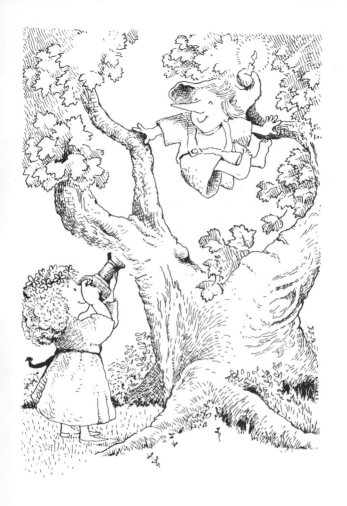

27.

Now and then, work out with a fitness expert to bring out your full potential. Afterward, practice by yourself to foster individual creativity. Think of your fitness work as artwork.

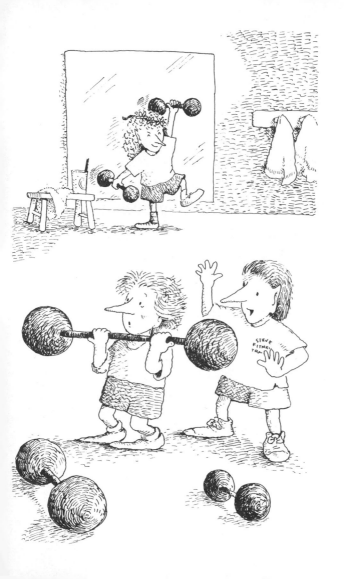

28.

Fitness training improves not only your physical well-being but also your determination. You are developing inner strength in addition to outer strength.

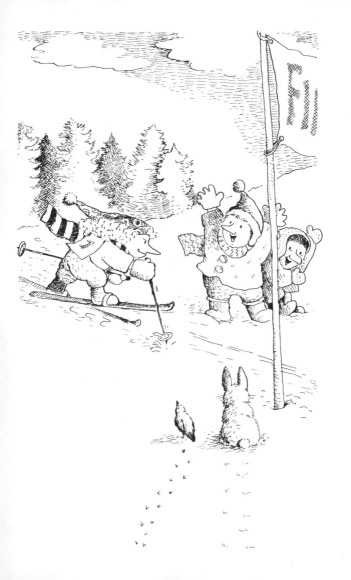

29.

Staying physically fit means actively enjoying the universe playing inside and all around you. Participate fully in this play.

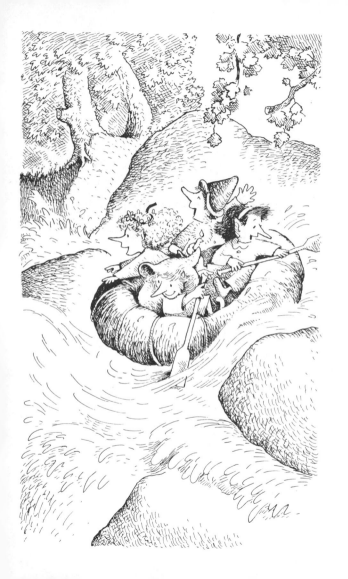

30.

Your physical condition can be a letter from your unconscious. When your body shows signs of stress, strain, or dis-ease, pay attention. Your unconscious may be warning you that your life is out of balance.

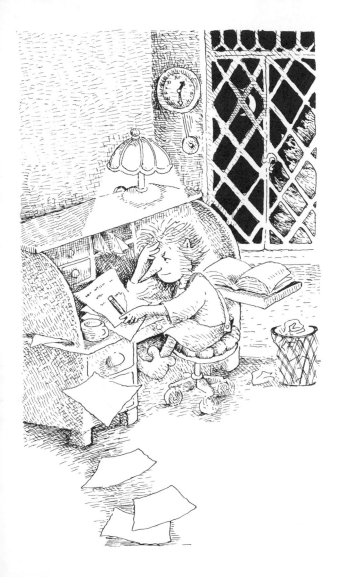

31.

Give your body the best, and it will give you its best. When your body is failing you in some way, consider if you have failed to honor its needs for healthful rest, diet, and exercise.

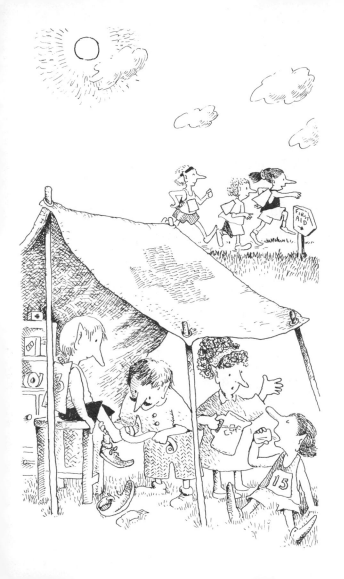

32.

Just as a plant thrives on water and the caress of sunlight, so your body thrives on touch and warming up to other bodies. Give and get some hugs each day.

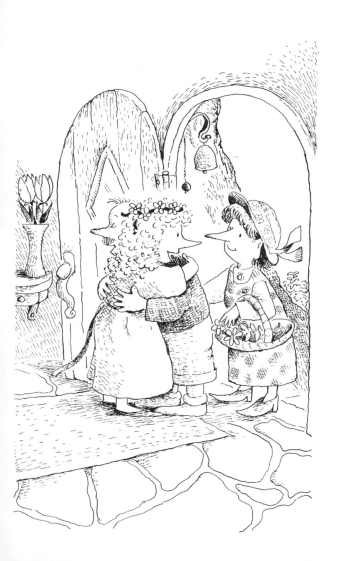

33.

Positive thinking is a healthy tonic. Think well of yourself. Think yourself well.

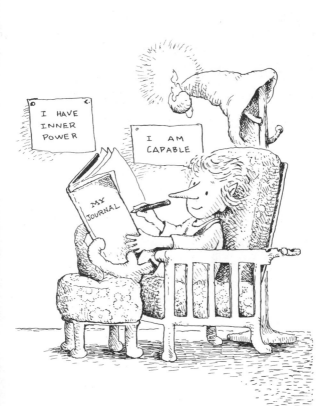

34.

Play out your fitness everywhere. This moment is your chance to empower and transform your body.

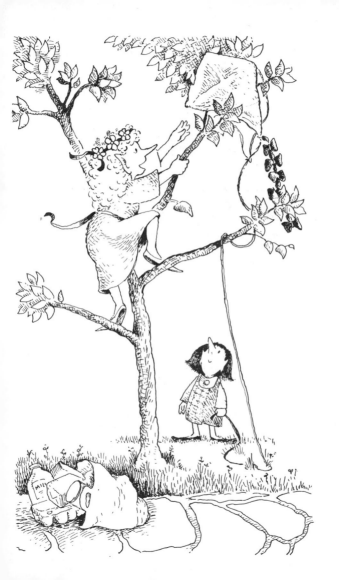

35.

Don't just <u>do</u> fitness; <u>be</u> it. Fitness is a natural expression of inner joy.

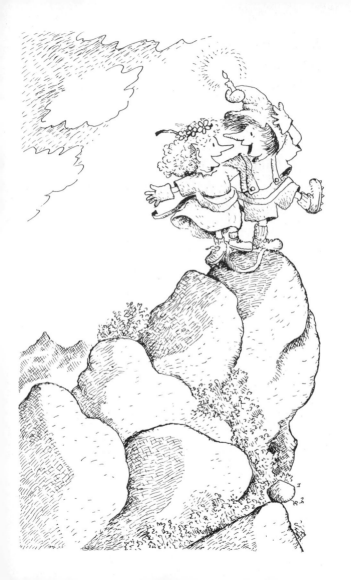

Steve Ilg is a nationally recognized multi-sport athlete and instructor of holistic fitness. He has written books and magazine articles. He lives in Durango, Colorado.

Illustrator for the Abbey Press Elf-help Books, **R.W. Alley** also illustrates and writes children's books. He lives in Barrington, Rhode Island, with his wife, daughter, and son.

The Story of the Abbey Press Elves

The engaging figures that populate the Abbey Press "elf-help" line of publications and products first appeared in 1987 on the pages of a small self-help book called *Be-good-to-yourself Therapy*. Shaped by the publishing staff's vision and defined in R.W. Alley's inventive illustrations, they lived out author Cherry Hartman's gentle, self-nurturing advice with charm, poignancy, and humor.

Reader response was so enthusiastic that more Elf-help Books were soon under way, a still-growing series that has inspired a line of related gift products.

The especially endearing character featured in the early books—sporting a cap with a mood-changing candle in its peak—has since been joined by a spirited female elf with flowers in her hair.

These two exuberant, sensitive, resourceful, kindhearted, lovable sprites, along with their lively elfin community, reveal what's truly important as they offer messages of joy and wonder, playfulness and co-creation, wholeness and serenity, the miracle of life and the mystery of God's love.

With wisdom and whimsy, these little creatures with long noses demonstrate the elf-help way to a rich and fulfilling life.

Elf-help Books...adding "a little character" and a lot of help to self-help reading!

Anger Therapy (new, improved binding)
#20127-7 $4.95   ISBN 0-87029-292-7

Caregiver Therapy (new, improved binding)
#20164-0 $4.95   ISBN 0-87029-285-4

Self-esteem Therapy (new, improved binding)
#20165-7 $4.95   ISBN 0-87029-280-3

Take-charge-of-your-life Therapy
   (new, improved binding)
#20168-1 $4.95   ISBN 0-87029-271-4

Work Therapy (new, improved binding)
#20166-5 $4.95   ISBN 0-87029-276-5

Everyday-courage Therapy
#20167-3 $3.95   ISBN 0-87029-274-9

Peace Therapy
#20176-4 $3.95   ISBN 0-87029-273-0

Friendship Therapy
#20174-9 $3.95   ISBN 0-87029-270-6

Christmas Therapy (color edition)
#20175-6 $5.95   ISBN 0-87029-268-4

Grief Therapy (new, improved binding)
#20178-0 $4.95   ISBN 0-87029-267-6

More Be-good-to-yourself Therapy
#20180-6 $3.95   ISBN 0-87029-262-5

Happy Birthday Therapy (new, improved binding)
#20181-4 $4.95   ISBN 0-87029-260-9

Forgiveness Therapy (new, improved binding)
#20184-8 $4.95   ISBN 0-87029-258-7

Keep-life-simple Therapy
#20185-5 $3.95   ISBN 0-87029-257-9